Super easy Plant-Based Cookbook

Super easy and delicious Plant-Based recipes to learn how to lose weight and feel fit!

Carolyn J. Perez

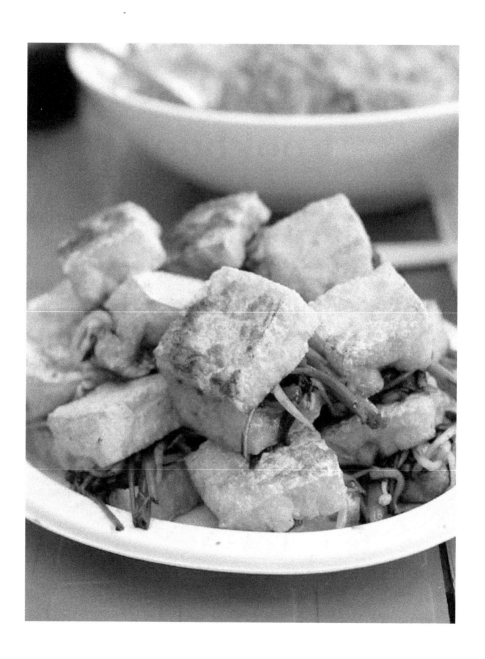

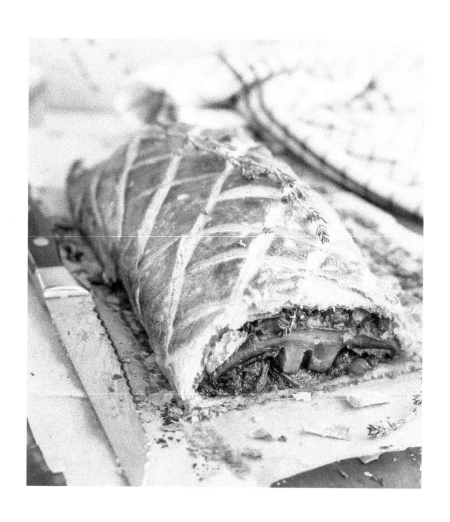

Contents

Introduction

It is a common thought to think that following a diet is necessarily linked to the concept of actual weight loss. However, this is not always the case: following a diet is often directly linked to the foods that we decide to include in our tables daily.

In addition, we do not always choose the best quality ingredients to cook our dishes.

Sometimes we are so rushed and unruly that we forget that we love our bodies. And what better cure than a healthy diet? Following a healthy diet should become more than an imposition or a punishment, but a real lifestyle.

Moreover, this is the Plant-based diet goal: not to impose a restrictive and sometimes impossible diet to follow, but to recreate a diet based on foods of natural origin and above all healthy. Therefore, the plant based represents a real food trend. However, as we will see it is much more than just a fashion trend, but a real lifestyle.

In addition, it is the aim of this text, or rather of this cookbook, to introduce you to the plant based discipline. And we will do it with a few theoretical explanations, just to make you understand what we are talking about and above all how to prepare it: there will be a purely practical part where you will find 800 recipes on the plant based. These recipes will be divided into appetizers, snacks, first and second courses, side dishes and finally a string of plant based desserts.

In the end, you will be spoiled for choice to start following this healthy dietary discipline.

Plant based diet: what are we talking about?

We already mentioned that more than a real weight loss diet the Plant based diet is a food discipline. Food discipline is enjoying great success not only because it is very fashionable, but because it applies such principles that can be perfectly integrated into our daily lives. The plant-based diet is a true approach to life, starting with nutrition: respect for one's health and body, first of all, which is reflected in respect for all forms of life and the planet in general. As the word itself says, it deals with a food plan based, precisely on what comes from plants. However, simply calling it that way would be too simplistic.

It is a predominantly plant-based diet, but not only. It is not just about consuming vegetables but about taking natural foods: not industrially processed, not treated, and not deriving from the exploitation of resources and animals, preferably zero km.

So it could be a discipline that aims not only at environmental saving but also at the economic one: think about what advantages, in fact, at the level of your pockets you can have if you apply the principle of 0Km and therefore to be able to harvest your vegetables directly from your garden.

Environmental savings do not only mean pollution reduction: the ethical component (present exclusively in the vegan diet, for example) is combined with a strong will to health. This means that the plant based, in addition to not preferring foods that exploit animals, is also based on foods that are especially unprocessed, fresh, healthy, balanced, light, and rich in essential nutrients. In practice, it is a plant-based diet but not vegan / vegetarian, emphasizing the quality and wholesomeness of foods rather than on their moral value, albeit with great attention to sustainability.

Such a lifestyle could therefore be of help, not only to our health, but also to create a more sustainable world for future generations.

Main differences between Vegan and Plant based diet

The plant-based diet is often associated with the vegan diet. This is because both plan to include cruelty free foods that do not involve any animal exploitation.

Furthermore, they are associated precisely because they are both predominantly plant-based.

However, there are some pretty obvious differences between these two diets.

First of all, precisely for the reasoning behind the prevalence of plants.

It is well known that even the vegan diet provides a diet based on foods of plant origin: unlike the plant-based diet, however, nothing of animal derivation is allowed, neither direct nor indirect, nor other products - clothing or accessories - which include the exploitation of animals.

No eggs, no milk, no honey, no leather, so to speak, and not only: in its most rigorous meanings, veganism does not even include the use of yeasts, as the bacteria that compose them are indisputably living beings.

A vegan diet can be balanced if the person who leads it knows well the foods and their combinations, the necessary supplements, and their body's reaction to the lack of certain foods.

On the contrary, the Plant-Based diet is on the one hand more relaxed, on the other more stringent.

What does it mean?

This means that it is on the one hand more relaxed because it is plant-based, but not exclusively vegetable: products of animal origin are allowed, in moderate quantities, but under only one condition, namely the excellent quality of the food itself and its certified origin. For example, eggs can be consumed occasionally but only if very fresh, possibly at zero km, from free-range farms where the hens are not exploited but can live outdoors without constraints.

It is also a somewhat more stringent philosophy than veganism precisely for this reason: as long as it is 100% vegetable, the vegan also consumes heavily processed foods, such as industrial fries. Therefore, the vegan can also eat junk foods or snacks. Conversely, plant-based dieters would never admit highly refined foods of this type.

Both dietary approaches are conscious and do not involve the consumption of meat. However, if vegans are driven by ethical reasons, those who follow a plant-based diet also reject everything processed on an industrial level and unhealthy.

A plant-based diet is a diet that aims to eliminate industrially processed foods and, therefore, potentially more harmful to health. It is based on the consumption of fruit and vegetables, whole grains and avoiding (or minimizing) animal products and processed foods. This means that vegan desserts made with refined sugar or bleached flour are also covered.

There is also a substantial difference between the philosophies behind the two diets. As we said in the previous paragraph and above, the ethical component, which is based on the refusal of any food of animal origin, plays a lot in veganism. While for the plant based is not a purely moral and moralistic discourse but on the real thought of being able to keep healthy with the food discipline and be respectful of the environment surrounding us.

Plant based diet full shopping list. What to eat and what to avoid

Now we can examine the complete shopping list of the plant based diet.
Let's briefly summarize the principles on which this particular type of diet is based:

- Emphasizes whole, minimally processed foods.
- Limits or avoids animal products.
- Focuses on plants, including vegetables, fruits, whole grains, legumes, seeds and nuts, which should make up most of what you eat.
- Excludes refined foods, like added sugars, white flour and processed oils.
- Pays special attention to food quality, promoting locally sourced, organic food whenever possible.

As for what you can usually eat, we can say the general consumption of:

- Wholegrain and flours
- extra virgin olive oil

- Seasonal fruit and vegetables: these foods are the basis of every meal.
- In this diet you can also eat sweets but only and exclusively homemade and with controlled raw materials, simple and not very refined, preferably of vegetable origin - for example by replacing milk with soy or rice drinks, and eggs with other natural thickeners such as flaxseed, or simple ripe banana.
- You can also consume nuts and seeds.

As for absolutely forbidden foods, there are all those ready-made and processed:

- ready-made sauces
- chips
- biscuits
- various kinds of snacks
- sugary cereals,
- Spreads, snacks and many other notoriously unhealthy foods.
- Junk food and fast food are therefore absolutely banned

- Sugar beverages

Regarding the complete shopping list:

- Fruits: Berries, citrus fruits, pears, peaches, pineapple, bananas, etc.
- Vegetables: Kale, spinach, tomatoes, broccoli, cauliflower, carrots, asparagus, peppers, etc.
- Starchy vegetables: Potatoes, sweet potatoes, butternut squash, etc.
- Whole grains: Brown rice, rolled oats, spelt, quinoa, brown rice pasta, barley, etc.
- Healthy fats with omega 3: Avocados, olive oil, coconut oil, unsweetened coconut, etc.
- Legumes: Peas, chickpeas, lentils, peanuts, beans, black beans, etc.
- Seeds, nuts and nut butter: Almonds, cashews, macadamia nuts, pumpkin seeds, sunflower seeds, natural peanut butter, tahini, etc.
- Unsweetened plant-based milk: Coconut milk, almond milk, cashew milk, etc.
- Spices, herbs and seasonings: Basil, rosemary, turmeric, curry, black pepper, salt, etc.

- Condiments: Salsa, mustard, nutritional yeast, soy sauce, vinegar, lemon juice, etc.
- Plant-based protein: Tofu, tempeh, seitan, and plant based protein sources or powders with no added sugar or artificial ingredients.
- Beverages: Coffee, tea, sparkling water, etc.

There is the chance to add food of animal origin very rarely, for example if you have specific nutritional needs or if it has been strongly recommended by your doctor. Anyway, if supplementing your plant-based diet with animal products choose quality products from grocery stores or, better yet, purchase them from local farms.

- Eggs: Pasture-raised when possible.
- Poultry: Free-range, organic when possible.
- Beef and pork: Pastured or grass-fed when possible.
- Seafood: Wild-caught from sustainable fisheries when possible.
- Dairy: Organic dairy products from pasture-raised animals whenever possible.

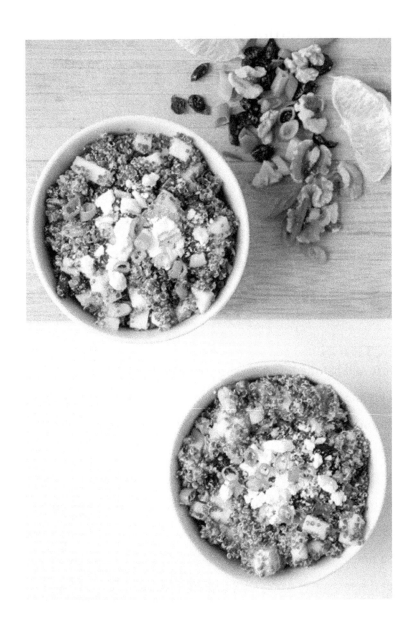

RECIPES

Tofu and almond meatballs

PREPARATION TIME: 20 minutes
COOKING TIME: 5 minutes
CALORIES: 263

INGREDIENTS FOR 4 SERVINGS

- 500 grams of tofu

- 40 grams of already skinned almonds

- Soy sauce to taste

- White sesame seeds to taste

- Olive oil to taste

- Salt and pepper to taste

DIRECTIONS

1. Rinse and pat the tofu with absorbent paper.

2. Cut it into cubes and sauté it in a pan with olive oil for 5 minutes.

3. Season with salt and pepper, stir and then turn off.

4. Now put the tofu in a bowl.

5. Mash the tofu with a fork. Now add the soy sauce and mix well.

6. Chop the almonds and then put them in the bowl with the tofu.

7. Mix well and then form meatballs by taking a little of the mixture at a time.

8. Put the sesame in a non-stick pan and toast it.

9. Now put the sesame on a plate and pass over the tofu balls.

10. The tofu meatballs are ready, put them on the plates and serve.

Seitan, avocado and tomatoes

PREPARATION TIME: 15 minutes

COOKING TIME: 6 minutes
CALORIES: 599

INGREDIENTS FOR 4 SERVINGS

- 500 grams of seitan
- 4 tomatoes
- 4 avocados
- 40 grams of cashews
- 8 mint leaves
- Olive oil to taste
- Salt and pepper to taste

DIRECTIONS

1. Wash the tomatoes and then cut them into cubes.
2. Peel and wash the avocado, remove the stone and cut the pulp into cubes.
3. Coarsely chop the cashews.
4. Wash and dry the mint leaves and then chop them. Put them in a bowl covered with oil and set aside.
5. Rinse and pat the seitan with absorbent paper and then cut it into slices.
6. Heat a grill and grill the slices of seitan 3 minutes per side.
7. Arrange the seitan on serving plates and garnish them with the

tomatoes and avocado.

8. Season with salt and pepper and then season with mint oil and serve.

Sandwiches with seitan, avocado and cucumbers

PREPARATION TIME: 20 minutes

COOKING TIME: 5 minutes

CALORIES: 578

INGREDIENTS FOR 4 SERVINGS

- 12 slices of wholemeal bread
- 4 small avocados
- 200 grams of seitan
- Half a cucumber
- 8 tablespoons of plant based mayonnaise
- Olive oil to taste
- Salt and pepper to taste

DIRECTIONS

1. Peel and wash the avocados. Remove the stone and then cut them into slices.
2. Put the avocado in a bowl and mash it with a fork.
3. Season it with oil, salt, pepper, and mix.
4. Dab the seitan with absorbent paper and then cut it into cubes.
5. Put it in a pan with hot oil and sauté for 5 minutes.
6. Season with salt and pepper and turn off. Put the seitan in a bowl and mash it with a fork.

7. Take a slice of bread and spread with avocado. Put the other slice of bread on top and spread the mayonnaise first and then the seitan. Close with another slice of bread.

8. Repeat the same operation for the other sandwiches.

9. Put on plates and serve.

Tempeh in saffron sauce

PREPARATION TIME: 15 minutes
COOKING TIME: 15 minutes

CALORIES: 390

INGREDIENTS FOR 4 SERVINGS

- 500 grams of tempeh
- 4 sage leaves
- 1 teaspoon of thyme leaves
- 100 grams of soy butter
- 2 sachets of saffron
- 2 tablespoons of oat flour
- 500 ml of vegetable broth
- Salt and pepper to taste

DIRECTIONS

1. Wash the sage leaves.
2. Dab the tempeh with absorbent paper and then cut it into cubes.
3. In a saucepan, melt the butter.
4. As soon as it has melted, add the flour, salt, pepper and saffron.
5. Mix well and as soon as the stone marten is well toasted, add the vegetable broth.
6. Cook until the sauce has thickened, stirring constantly.
7. Now put a tablespoon of oil in a pan.
8. Let it heat up and then put the tempeh to sauté for 5 minutes.

9.   Season with salt and pepper and add the sauce.

10. Stir, cook for a couple of minutes and turn off.

11. Put on plates and serve.

Tofu with tomato

PREPARATION TIME: 15 minutes
COOKING TIME: 25 minutes
CALORIES: 239

INGREDIENTS FOR 4 SERVINGS

- 200 ml of tomato sauce
- 1 onion
- 1 clove of garlic
- 500 grams of tofu
- 200 ml of vegetable broth
- 1 teaspoon of oregano
- Salt and pepper to taste
- Olive oil to taste

DIRECTIONS

1. Rinse and pat the tofu and then cut it into cubes.
2. Peel the garlic and onion and chop them.
3. Put a tablespoon of olive oil in a pan and then put the garlic and onion to fry.
4. After a couple of minutes, add the tomato sauce.
5. Season with salt and pepper, stir and brown for 2 minutes.
6. Now add the vegetable broth and cook for 15 minutes.
7. Now add the tofu cubes and continue cooking for another 5 minutes.

8. After 5 minutes, turn off and sprinkle with oregano.

9. Stir, season well then put on plates and serve.

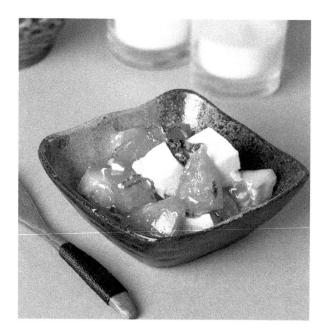

Tofu with honey and cinnamon

PREPARATION TIME: 15 minutes+30 minutes to rest

COOKING TIME: 20minutes

CALORIES: 297

INGREDIENTS FOR 4 SERVINGS

- 600 grams of tofu
- 80 ml of honey
- 150 ml of vegetable broth
- 1 tablespoon of ground cinnamon
- 2 tablespoons of olive oil

DIRECTIONS

1. Rinse and pat the tofu with absorbent paper then cut it into cubes.
2. Put it in a large enough bowl.
3. Mix the honey with the oil and vegetable broth in another bowl.
4. Add the cinnamon and mix until you get a homogeneous emulsion.
5. Pour the emulsion over the tofu and leave to marinate for 30 minutes.
6. After 30 minutes, transfer the tofu with the marinade in a pan.
7. Cook the tofu until the liquid has reduced by half.
8. Turn off, put on serving plates and serve immediately.

Sautéed tofu with herbs

PREPARATION TIME: 15 minutes
COOKING TIME: 10minutes

CALORIES: 174

INGREDIENTS FOR 4 SERVINGS

- 400 grams of tofu
- 1 tablespoon of chopped chives
- 1 tablespoon of curry powder
- 1 teaspoon of ground ginger
- 1 sprig of chopped parsley
- Salt and pepper to taste
- Olive oil to taste

DIRECTIONS

1. Rinse and pat the tofu with absorbent paper, then cut it into cubes.
2. Heat a tablespoon of oil in a pan and as soon as it is hot, add the chives, curry, ginger and parsley.
3. Cook for a minute, stirring constantly.
4. Now add the tofu cubes and mix.
5. Sauté for 5 minutes, then season with salt and pepper.
6. Stir one last time, and then turn off.
7. Put the tofu on the plates and serve.

Quiche with spinach and plant based ricotta

PREPARATION TIME: 10 minutes
COOKING TIME: 40 minutes

CALORIES: 428

INGREDIENTS FOR 4 SERVINGS

- 500 grams of spinach
- 350 grams of plant based ricotta
- 300 grams of plant based puff pastry
- 1 plant based mozzarella
- 1 clove of garlic
- 1 teaspoon of nutmeg
- Salt and pepper to taste
- Olive oil to taste

DIRECTIONS

1. Carefully wash the spinach and then let it drain.
2. Peel and wash the garlic and then chop it.
3. Put a tablespoon of oil in a saucepan and then brown the garlic.
4. Now add the spinach, season with salt and pepper and cook for 10 minutes.
5. After 10 minutes, drain and then chop.
6. Put them in a bowl and add the ricotta and diced mozzarella and nutmeg.
7. Stir to flavour well.
8. Brush a pan with olive oil and line it with the puff pastry.

9. Pour the ricotta, spinach mixture inside, and put in the oven.

10. Cook for 30 minutes at 180 ° C.

11. As soon as it is cooked, take it out of the oven and let it rest for 5 minutes.

12. Now cut into slices, put the quiche on the plates and serve.

Chickpea and olive salad

PREPARATION TIME: 10 minutes
COOKING TIME: 1 hour and 30 minutes

CALORIES: 490

INGREDIENTS FOR 4 SERVINGS

- 200 grams of chickpeas already soaked
- 150 grams of green olives
- 150 grams of black olives
- 10 mint leaves
- 1 sprig of thyme
- 1 shallot
- 1 lemon
- Salt and pepper to taste
- Olive oil to taste

DIRECTIONS

1. Wash and dry the thyme and mint leaves.
2. Chop the mint leaves.
3. Put the chickpeas and thyme in a pan covered with water.
4. Cover the pot with a lid and cook for 1 hour and 30 minutes.
5. After the cooking time, season with salt and pepper, stir and then turn off.
6. Drain the chickpeas, put them in a salad bowl and add the olives.
7. Wash and dry the lemon, cut it in half.
8. Squeeze one-half on the chickpeas and cut the other half into

slices.

9. Put the lemon slices in the salad bowl with the chickpeas.

10. Sprinkle with the chopped mint leaves. Season with oil, salt and pepper, mix and serve.

Chickpea and tofu salad

PREPARATION TIME: 30 minutes
CALORIES: 154

INGREDIENTS FOR 4 SERVINGS
- 300 grams of cooked chickpeas
- 1 zucchini
- 1 shallot
- 60 grams of tofu
- 1 lemon
- 1 yellow pepper
- 100 grams of cherry tomatoes
- 1 small cucumber
- 4 mint leaves
- Olive oil to taste
- Salt and Pepper To Taste.

DIRECTIONS
1. Remove the cap from the pepper, cut it in half, remove the seeds and white filaments and then wash it. Cut it into strips.
2. Peel and wash the shallot and then cut it into slices.
3. Wash the zucchini and then cut it into slices.
4. Wash the cherry tomatoes and cut them in half.
5. Wash the cucumber and cut it into slices.
6. Put the vegetables in a salad bowl and add the chickpeas.
7. Rinse and pat the tofu with absorbent paper.

8. Heat a grill and when hot, grill the tofu, 3 minutes per side.

9. Remove the tofu from the grill and cut it into cubes. Put the tofu in the salad bowl with the chickpeas and vegetables.

10. In a bowl put the lemon juice, two tablespoons of olive oil, salt and pepper and mix everything with a fork.

11. Dress the salad with the emulsion, mix to flavour everything well and serve.

Broccoli and spelt salad

PREPARATION TIME: 25 minutes
COOKING TIME: 15 minutes
CALORIES: 233

INGREDIENTS FOR 4 SERVINGS

- 120 grams of spelt
- 50 grams of chopped walnuts
- 8 black olives
- 300 grams of broccoli flowers
- 4 cherry tomatoes
- Olive oil to taste
- Salt and Pepper To Taste.

DIRECTIONS

1. Start by preparing the spelt. Rinse it under running water and cook it in boiling salted water for 15 minutes.

2. Meanwhile, wash the broccoli flowers and then put them to boil in another pot, for 10 minutes, in boiling salted water.

3. As soon as the broccoli is cooked, drain it, put it on a cutting board and cut it into small pieces. Put them in a salad bowl.

4. Wash the cherry tomatoes and cut them in half.

5. Put the olives and cherry tomatoes in the salad bowl with the broccoli.

6. As soon as the spelt is cooked, drain it and then put it in the salad

bowl.

7. Season with oil, salt and pepper and mix well.

8. Sprinkle with chopped walnuts and serve.

Broad bean and tofu salad

PREPARATION TIME: 40 minutes
COOKING TIME: 10 minutes
CALORIES: 165

INGREDIENTS FOR 4 SERVINGS

- 800 grams of fresh beans already peeled
- 40 grams of tofu
- 2 tablespoons of balsamic vinegar
- The zest of one lemon
- Olive oil to taste
- Salt and pepper to taste

DIRECTIONS

1. Wash and then drain the beans.
2. Bring a pot of water and salt to a boil and cook the beans for 5 minutes.
3. After 15 minutes, drain the beans and let them cool.
4. Meanwhile, rinse and pat the tofu with paper towels, then cut into cubes.
5. Put a tablespoon of olive oil in a pan and as soon as it is hot enough, sauté the tofu for 3 minutes.
6. Wash the lemon zest and then cut it into slices. Put it in a bowl and add a tablespoon of olive oil, salt, pepper and balsamic vinegar and mix with a fork.

7. Now put the broad beans in a salad bowl together with the tofu.

8. Sprinkle with the emulsion, mix and serve.

Quinoa and zucchini salad

PREPARATION TIME: 30 minutes
COOKING TIME: 25 minutes
CALORIES: 543

INGREDIENTS FOR 4 SERVINGS

- 480 grams of quinoa
- 4 zucchinis
- 2 shallots
- 4 sheets of nori seaweed
- 2 tablespoons of sesame seeds
- 2 cloves of garlic
- Soy sauce to taste
- Olive oil to taste
- Salt and Pepper To Taste.

DIRECTIONS

1. Rinse the quinoa and let it drain.
2. Bring the water to a boil with the salt and put the quinoa to cook for 15 minutes.
3. Meanwhile, wash the zucchinis and cut them into cubes.
4. Peel and wash the shallots and cut them into slices.
5. Peel and wash the garlic cloves.
6. Put the garlic and shallots to brown in a pan with a tablespoon of olive oil.
7. As soon as they are golden brown, add the zucchinis.

8. Stir and then add a tablespoon of soy sauce.

9. Season with salt, pepper, and sauté for 5 minutes.

10. Drain the quinoa and place it in the pan with the zucchini.

11. Stir, season with salt, pepper, and cook for another 10 minutes.

12. Remove from the heat, pour the zucchini and quinoa into a salad bowl, and let it cool.

13. As soon as they are cold, add the nori t seaweed

Mixed salad with chopped hazelnuts

PREPARATION TIME: 15 minutes
CALORIES: 200

INGREDIENTS FOR 4 SERVINGS

- 1 cooked beetroot
- 1 cooked yellow beet
- 4 radishes
- 2 carrots
- 1 orange
- 1 lemon
- 4 tablespoons of chopped walnuts
- Olive oil to taste
- Salt and pepper to taste

DIRECTIONS

1. Peel the two beets and then cut them into slices.
2. Peel and wash the carrots and then cut them into slices.
3. Wash the radishes and cut them into slices.
4. In a bowl, combine the lemon juice, orange juice, 4 tablespoons of olive oil, salt and pepper. Stir with a fork until you get a homogeneous emulsion.
5. Now put the radishes, beets and carrots on a plate.
6. Dress them with the emulsion and then sprinkle the surface with chopped hazelnuts.
7. You can serve.

Quinoa stuffed peppers

PREPARATION TIME: 30 minutes

COOKING TIME: 1 hour
CALORIES: 183

INGREDIENTS FOR 4 SERVINGS

- 4 medium-sized red peppers

- 100 grams of quinoa

- 100 grams of soy cheese

- 200 ml of vegetable broth

- A tablespoon of chopped chives

- Two sprigs of chopped parsley

- A spoonful of poppy seeds

- Olive oil to taste

- Salt and Pepper To Taste.

DIRECTIONS

1. Start by making the quinoa. Put the vegetable broth in a saucepan and bring to a boil.

2. Put the quinoa in the boiling broth and cook for 15 minutes.

3. After 15 minutes turn off, put the lid on the pot and let it rest for 5 minutes.

4. Meanwhile, remove the cap from the peppers and wash them.

5. Remove the internal seeds and leave the peppers whole.

6. Sprinkle the peppers with salt and pepper and then place them in a pan brushed with olive oil.

7. Now put the quinoa in a bowl. Add the soy cheese cut into small pieces, poppy seeds, parsley, chives, and oil, salt, pepper, and mix well to flavour everything.

8. Put the quinoa mixture inside the peppers. Sprinkle the surface

9. with a drizzle of oil and bake in the oven at 180 ° C for 40 minutes.

Seitan baked in foil with broccoli and carrots

PREPARATION TIME: 10 minutes
COOKING TIME: 15 minutes
CALORIES: 220

INGREDIENTS FOR 4 SERVINGS

- 400 grams of seitan

- 4 carrots

- 24 broccoli flowers

- Salt and Pepper to taste

- Olive oil to taste

DIRECTIONS

1. Peel and wash the carrots and then cut them into thin slices.

2. Wash the broccoli flowers and then cut them into small pieces.

3. Rinse the seitan and pat it dry with absorbent paper. Cut it into slices.

4. Take 4 aluminium foil and put the carrots at the bottom of the foil.

5. Season them with oil, salt, and pepper and then add the seitan.

6. Season the seitan with oil, salt and pepper and finally add the broccoli and season them in the same way.

7. Close the aluminium foil and place them inside an oven pan.

8. Put the pan in the oven and cook for 15 minutes at 180 ° C.

9. As soon as the cooking time has passed, remove the pan from the oven, open the packets and let it evaporate for a couple of minutes.

10. Put the foil on the serving plates and serve.

Zucchini stuffed with quinoa and tofu

PREPARATION TIME: 25 minutes

COOKING TIME: 20 minutes
CALORIES: 200

INGREDIENTS FOR 4 SERVINGS

- 4 zucchinis
- 240 grams of cooked quinoa
- 120 grams of tofu
- 2 tablespoons of capers
- 8 green olives
- 6 cherry tomatoes
- Salt and Pepper To Taste.
- Olive oil to taste

DIRECTIONS

1. Wash the zucchinis and then cut them in half lengthwise.
2. With the help of a spoon, scoop out the pulp and put it in the blender glass.
3. Wash the cherry tomatoes and cut them in half.
4. Cut the olives in half and remove the stone.
5. Dab the tofu with absorbent paper and then cut it into cubes.
6. Put the cherry tomatoes, tofu and olives in the glass of the blender.
7. Add two tablespoons of oils, salt, pepper, and blend everything at

maximum speed for a couple of minutes.

8. Put the mixture in a bowl and add the quinoa and mix.

9. Brush a baking sheet with a little oil and put the zucchini inside.

10. Fill the zucchinis with the quinoa mixture and place in the oven.

11. Cook at 200 ° C for 20 minutes.

12. As soon as they are cooked, let them cool slightly and then serve.

Seitan steaks with curry sauce and pine nuts

PREPARATION TIME: 7 minutes
COOKING TIME: 13 minutes
CALORIES: 312

INGREDIENTS FOR 4 SERVINGS

- 400 grams of seitan
- 2 leeks
- 20 grams of pine nuts
- 70 grams of soy butter
- 100 ml of vegetable broth
- 1 teaspoon of curry
- 2 tablespoons of coconut milk
- 10 strands of chopped chives
- Salt and pepper to taste
- Olive oil to taste

DIRECTIONS

1. Remove the green part and the hardest leaves of the leeks, wash them and cut them into slices.
2. Rinse the seitan, pat it dry with absorbent paper and cut it into slices.
3. Put the coconut milk in a bowl and add the curry. Stir until the two ingredients are well blended.
4. Put the butter in a pan. Let it melt and then put the leeks to sauté for 5 minutes, stirring often.

5. Now add the broth, stir and cook for 2 minutes for sides.

6. Add the milk to the curry and continue cooking for another 5 minutes over low heat. Season with salt, pepper, and then turn off.

7. Prepare the seitan now. Heat a little oil in a pan and as soon as it is hot, cook the seitan for three minutes per side.

8. Now add the curry sauce, cook for a couple of minutes and turn off.

9. Transfer the slices of seitan to plates. Sprinkle them with the curry sauce, pine nuts and chopped chives and serve.

Tempeh fillets with spicy sauce

PREPARATION TIME: 20 minutes
COOKING TIME: 5 minutes
CALORIES: 280

INGREDIENTS FOR 4 SERVINGS

- 400 grams of tempeh
- A clove of garlic
- 10 green olives
- 100 grams of tomato pulp
- A chili pepper
- Olive oil to taste
- Salt and pepper to taste

DIRECTIONS

1. Peel and wash the garlic clove.
2. Rinse the tempeh and pat it dry with absorbent paper. Cut it into slices.
3. Wash the chilli and then cut it into small pieces.
4. Cut the olives in half, remove the stone and then chop them.
5. Heat a tablespoon of oil in a pan and as soon as it is hot, brown the garlic.
6. Put the tempeh, cook it for 3 minutes and then remove it and set it aside.
7. Now put the chopped olives, the tomato pulp and the chilli pepper in the same pan.

8. Cook for 2 minutes, stirring to flavour well.

9. Now put the tempeh back in the pan. Season with salt and pepper, stir and continue cooking for another minute.

10. Turn off and put the tempeh on serving plates. Sprinkle with the sauce and serve.

Seitan morsels with pear sauce

PREPARATION TIME: 20 minutes

COOKING TIME: 30 minutes
CALORIES: 320

INGREDIENTS FOR 4 SERVINGS

- 400 grams of seitan
- 300 grams of pears
- 100 ml of vegetable broth
- Half a lemon
- 30 grams of grated ginger
- 30 grams of soy butter
- Salt and pepper to taste

DIRECTIONS

1. Dab the seitan with absorbent paper and then cut it into cubes.
2. Peel the pears, remove the seeds, wash them and then cut them into cubes.
3. Put the pears in a saucepan, add the vegetable broth, and cook for 20 minutes.
4. After 20 minutes turn off and blend everything with an immersion blender.
5. Put the butter in a pan and as soon as it is melted, put the seitan cubes.
6. Cook them for 5 minutes, and then season with salt and pepper.

7. Now add the pear cream and ginger. Stir and cook for another 5 minutes.

8. In the meantime, wash and dry the lemon and cut it into rings.

9. Now put the seitan and the cream on the serving plates add the lemon slices and serve.

Plant based crepes with vegetables

PREPARATION TIME: 20 minutes
COOKING TIME: 30 minutes
CALORIES: 514

INGREDIENTS FOR 4 SERVINGS

- 4 plant based crepes

- 2 zucchinis

- 2 carrots

- 200 grams of pumpkin

- 1 onion

- 600 ml of plant based béchamel

- 2 plant based mozzarella

- Salt and Pepper To Taste.

- Olive oil to taste

DIRECTIONS

1. Wash the zucchinis and then cut them into cubes.

2. Peel and wash the carrots and then cut them into cubes.

3. Peel the pumpkin, remove the seeds, wash it and cut it into cubes.

4. Peel and wash the onion and then cut it into slices.

5. Put two tablespoons of oil in a pan and when hot, put the vegetables to sauté for 10 minutes.

6. Season with salt and pepper, mix and turn off.

7. Cut the mozzarella into cubes.

8. Now take a round baking pan and brush it with olive oil.

9. Place the first crepe and sprinkle it with the béchamel, spreading it with a spoon.

10. Put some vegetables on top, a few cubes of mozzarella and then cover with the other crepe.

11. Repeat the same operation until all the ingredients are used up.

12. Put in the oven and cook at 180 ° C for 20 minutes.

13. As soon as they are cooked, take them out of the oven and let them cool.

14. Now cut them into 4 portions, put them on plates and serve.

Wholemeal sandwich with vegetables

PREPARATION TIME: 15 minutes
COOKING TIME: 15 minutes
CALORIES: 261

INGREDIENTS FOR 4 SERVINGS

- 4 wholemeal round rolls
- 2 eggplants
- 4 zucchinis
- 3 tomatoes
- Olive oil to taste
- Salt and pepper to taste

DIRECTIONS

1. Wash the zucchinis and cut them into rings.
2. Wash the eggplants and cut them into slices.
3. Brush the zucchinis and eggplants with oil and sprinkle them with salt and pepper.
4. Heat a grill and put the zucchinis and eggplants to grill.
5. Put the cooked vegetables on a plate and temporarily set aside.
6. Meanwhile, wash the tomatoes and then cut them into slices.
7. Cut the sandwiches in half and then brush them with a little oil.
8. First, put the grilled vegetables inside and then the tomatoes and then close the sandwiches.
9. You can now serve.

Seitan with cumin, chili and lime

PREPARATION TIME: 15 minutes
COOKING TIME: 12 minutes

CALORIES: 387

INGREDIENTS FOR 4 SERVINGS

- 400 grams of seitan
- 1 tablespoon of cumin seeds
- 1 tablespoon of paprika powder
- 1 chilli
- 4 limes
- 40 ml of soy sauce
- Olive oil to taste
- Salt and pepper to taste

DIRECTIONS

1. Wash and dry the limes. Grate the zest and strain the juice into a bowl.
2. Add the lime zest, oil, salt, pepper and soy sauce to the bowl. Mix well.
3. Dab the seitan with absorbent paper. Put it in the bowl with the emulsion and turn it a couple of times.
4. Cover the bowl with transparent paper and put in the fridge to marinate for an hour.
5. Brush a baking pan with olive oil.

6. After the marinating time, drain the seitan and place it in the pan.

7. Wash the chilli and then chop it.

8. Sprinkle the seitan with the chilli, cumin seeds and paprika.

9. Season with the marinating liquid and put in the oven.

10. Cook at 200 ° C for 12 minutes.

11. After the cooking time, remove from the oven and cut the seitan into slices.

12. Put it on plates, sprinkle it with the cooking juices and serve.

Tofu and pineapple skewers

PREPARATION TIME: 15 minutes

COOKING TIME: 10 minutes
CALORIES: 248

INGREDIENTS FOR 4 SERVINGS
- 500 grams of pineapple
- 2 bananas
- 2 green peppers
- 100 grams of tofu
- Half a lemon
- 1 sprig of chopped parsley
- Salt and pepper to taste
- Olive oil to taste

DIRECTIONS
1. Start with the tofu. Rinse it and pat it dry with absorbent paper, then cut it into cubes.
2. Heat a tablespoon of oil in a pan and as soon as it is hot, sauté the tofu for 3-4 minutes.
3. Season with salt and pepper, add the juice of half a lemon, then turn off and set aside.
4. Wash and dry the peppers. Cut them in half. Remove the white filaments and seeds.
5. Now cut the peppers into thin slices.

6. Peel the bananas and then cut them into cubes.

7. Peel and wash the pineapple then cut the pulp into cubes.

8. Now start forming the skewers. Start with the tofu, then the pepper, then the banana and finally the pineapple.

9. Continue like this until all the ingredients are used up.

10. Take a baking pan and brush it with olive oil.

11. Place the skewers inside and season with oil, salt and pepper.

12. Cook at 200 ° C for 5 minutes.

13. After the cooking time, take them out of the oven. Put them on serving plates.

14. Sprinkle with the chopped parsley and serve.

Plant based quiche with mushrooms and ricotta

PREPARATION TIME: 20 minutes

COOKING TIME: 45 minutes
CALORIES: 399

INGREDIENTS FOR 4 SERVINGS

- 300 grams of plant based puff pastry
- 400 grams of champignon mushrooms
- 250 grams of plant based ricotta
- 20 grams of chopped walnuts
- 1 clove of garlic
- 1 sprig of chopped parsley
- Olive oil to taste
- Salt and pepper to taste

DIRECTIONS

1. Start with the mushrooms. Remove the earthy part, wash them, dry them and then cut them into slices.
2. Peel and wash the garlic and then chop it.
3. In a pan, heat a tablespoon of olive oil.
4. As soon as it is hot, put the garlic to brown.
5. Now add the mushrooms, season with salt and pepper and cook for 8 minutes.
6. When cooked, add the chopped parsley, mix and turn off.
7. Put the ricotta in a bowl. Add the chopped walnuts, salt, pepper,

and mix everything well.

8. Take a baking tray and brush it with olive oil. Line it with the puff pastry.

9. Put the ricotta filling inside the puff pastry.

10. Sprinkle the surface with the mushrooms and place the pan in the oven.

11. Cook at 175 ° C for 35 minutes.

12. As soon as it is cooked, take the quiche out of the oven and let it cool.

13. Now cut it into slices put it on plates and serve.

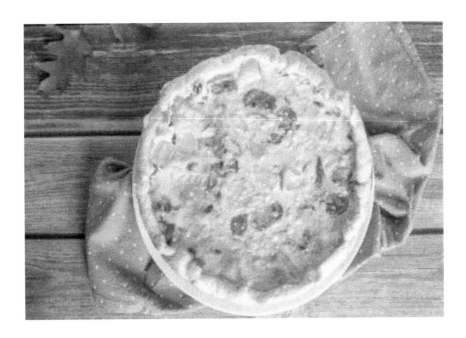

Quiche with olives and zucchinis

PREPARATION TIME: 20 minutes
COOKING TIME: 45 minutes
CALORIES: 480

INGREDIENTS FOR 4 SERVINGS

- 300 grams of plant based puff pastry

- 100 grams of black olives

- 1 tablespoon of capers

- 1 clove of garlic

- 500 grams of zucchinis

- 150 ml of soy cream

- Olive oil to taste

- Salt and pepper to taste

DIRECTIONS

1. Pitted the olives and put them in the glass of the mixer together with the capers.

2. Peel and wash the garlic and put it together with the olives.

3. Chop until you get a smooth and homogeneous mixture.

4. Wash the zucchinis and then grate them with a greater with large holes.

5. Heat a tablespoon of olive oil and as soon as it is hot, put the zucchinis to cook for 5 minutes. Season with salt and pepper and turn off.

6. Now put the cream in the pan with the zucchini and mix.

7. Brush a baking sheet and line it with the puff pastry.

8. Put the olive mixture at the bottom and then cover with the zucchini mixture.

9. Put the pan in the oven and cook at 200 ° C for 35 minutes.

10. After the cooking time, remove from the oven and let it cool.

11. Cut into slices, put on serving plates and serve.

Pumpkin, mushroom and potato pie

PREPARATION TIME: 20 minutes
COOKING TIME: 35 minutes

CALORIES: 264

INGREDIENTS FOR 4 SERVINGS

- 500 grams of pumpkin
- 500 grams of champignon mushrooms
- 400 grams of potatoes
- 200 grams of tomato pulp
- 1 teaspoon of oregano
- 1 plant based mozzarella
- 4 tablespoons of soy cream
- Olive oil to taste
- Salt and pepper to taste

DIRECTIONS

1. Start with the potatoes. Peel them, wash them and then cut them into thin slices.
2. Take an oven dish and brush it with olive oil.
3. Put the potatoes on the bottom and season with oil, salt and pepper.
4. Remove the earthy part from the mushrooms, rinse, dry them, and then cut them into thin slices.
5. Peel and remove the seeds from the pumpkin. Wash it and cut it

into slices.

6. Place the mushroom slices on top of the potatoes. Also, season the mushrooms with oil, salt and pepper.

7. Now put the pumpkin slices and season them with oil, salt and pepper.

8. Now put the tomato pulp and season with oil, salt and pepper.

9. Slice the mozzarella and put it on top of the tomato.

10. Sprinkle with oregano and put in the oven.

11. Cook at 180°C for 35 minutes.

12. After the cooking time, take the pie out of the oven and let it cool.

13. Now cut the pie into slices put it on plates and serve.

Zucchini stuffed with ricotta and mozzarella

PREPARATION TIME: 20 minutes

COOKING TIME: 45 minutes
CALORIES: 224

INGREDIENTS FOR 4 SERVINGS
* 6 zucchinis

* 200 grams of plant based ricotta

* 1 plant based mozzarella

* Salt and pepper to taste

* 1 teaspoon of nutmeg

* Olive oil to taste

DIRECTIONS
1. Wash the zucchinis and then put them to cook for 15 minutes in plenty of salted water.

2. Drain the courgettes and let them cool.

3. First cut them in half horizontally and then in half vertically.

4. With a spoon scoop out the pulp of the zucchini.

5. Sprinkle the remaining courgette with salt and pepper.

6. In a bowl, put together the ricotta, the diced mozzarella, salt, pepper and nutmeg.

7. Stir to flavour everything well.

8. Take a baking pan, brush it with olive oil and put the zucchini inside.

9. Fill the cavities of the zucchini with the ricotta and mozzarella mixture.

10. Sprinkle the surface with oil and then put in the oven at 180 ° C for 30 minutes.

11. As soon as they are cooked, take them out of the oven, put them on plates and serve immediately.

Quiche with broccoli

PREPARATION TIME: 20 minutes
COOKING TIME: 45 minutes
CALORIES: 380

INGREDIENTS FOR 4 SERVINGS

- 300 gr of plant based puff pastry

- 400 grams of broccoli flowers

- 350 grams of plant based ricotta

- 350 ml of soymilk

- Salt and pepper to taste

- Olive oil to taste

DIRECTIONS

1. Wash and then cut the broccoli flowers into small pieces.

2. Bring a pot of water and salt to a boil and then cook the broccoli for 5 minutes.

3. After 5 minutes, drain and let them cool.

4. Put the ricotta, milk, salt and pepper in a bowl and mix well.

5. Brush a pan with olive oil. Line it with the puff pastry.

6. Put the broccoli inside first and then the ricotta mixture.

7. Bake and cook at 200 ° C for 40 minutes.

8. As soon as it is cooked, take it out of the oven, let it cool and then cut it into slices.

9. Put the quiche on the plates and serve.

Quiche with spicy broccoli and stracchino

PREPARATION TIME: 20 minutes

COOKING TIME: 45 minutes
CALORIES: 380

INGREDIENTS FOR 4 SERVINGS

- 300 gr of plant based puff pastry (see basic recipe)
- 400 grams of broccoli flowers
- 350 grams of plant based stracchino (see basic recipe)
- 350 ml of soymilk
- Salt and pepper to taste
- 1 pinch of chilli powder
- 1 pinch of smoked paprika
- Olive oil to taste

DIRECTIONS

1. Wash and then cut the broccoli flowers into small pieces.
2. Bring a pot of water, chilli powder, paprika and salt to a boil and then cook the broccoli for 5 minutes.
3. After 5 minutes, drain and let them cool.
4. Put the stracchino, milk, salt and pepper in a bowl and mix well.
5. Brush a pan with olive oil. Line it with the puff pastry.
6. Put the broccoli inside first and then the ricotta mixture.
7. Bake and cook at 200 ° C for 40 minutes.
8. As soon as it is cooked, take it out of the oven, let it cool and then

cut it into slices.

9. Put the quiche on the plates and serve.

Seitan with potatoes and onions

PREPARATION TIME: 20 minutes
COOKING TIME: 25 minutes
CALORIES: 366

INGREDIENTS FOR 4 SERVINGS

- 400 grams of seitan

- 4 onions

- 12 medium sized potatoes

- 8 sage leaves

- Olive oil to taste

- Salt and pepper to taste

DIRECTIONS

1. Peel the potatoes, wash them thoroughly and then cut them into slices.

2. Peel and wash the onions and then slice them.

3. Rinse the seitan and then pat it dry with absorbent paper. Cut it into slices.

4. Put 2 tablespoons of olive oil in a pan and then put the onion to brown for a couple of minutes.

5. Add the potatoes, salt, pepper, and mix.

6. Cook for 15 minutes and then turn off.

7. Brush a baking sheet with oil and then put the potatoes and onions inside.

8. Put the seitan on top and season with oil, salt and pepper.

9. Put in the oven and cook at 200 ° C for 10 minutes.

10. After the cooking time, remove from the oven and let it rest for a couple of minutes.

11. Put the vegetables on the bottom of the plates first and then the seitan and serve.

Seitan with potatoes and onions

PREPARATION TIME: 15 minutes
COOKING TIME: 10 minutes
CALORIES: 298

INGREDIENTS FOR 4 SERVINGS

- 600 grams of seitan
- 10 sage leaves
- 200 ml of soymilk
- 50 grams of soy butter
- 20 grams of oat flour
- 2 tablespoons of soy sauce
- Salt and pepper to taste
- Olive oil to taste

DIRECTIONS

1. Dab the seitan with absorbent paper and then cut it into cubes.
2. Wash the sage and then chop it.
3. Melt the butter in a pan and then put the seitan to sauté.
4. Cook them for 5 minutes and then add the soy sauce.
5. Cook for a couple of minutes and then add the sage.
6. Continue for another 5 minutes and then add the flour and milk.
7. Stir constantly and continue cooking until the milk and flour have thickened.

8. Season with salt and pepper, stir one last time and turn off.

9. Put the seitan with the sauce on the serving plates and serve.

Tofu in maple syrup

PREPARATION TIME: 20 minutes+ 30 minutes to
   marinate
COOKING TIME: 10 minutes
CALORIES: 219

INGREDIENTS FOR 4 SERVINGS

- 400 grams of tofu
- 2 lemons
- 1 onion
- 2 cloves of garlic
- 3 sprigs of rosemary
- 2 tablespoons of maple syrup
- Olive oil to taste
- Salt and pepper to taste

DIRECTIONS

1. Rinse the tofu and then pat it dry with absorbent paper.
2. He put the tofu in a bowl.
3. Wash and dry the rosemary and place it in the bowl with the tofu.
4. Peel and wash the onion and garlic cloves and then chop them.
   Put them in the bowl with the tofu.
5. Squeeze and strain the lemon juice into the bowl with the tofu,
   add oil, salt, pepper and maple syrup.
6. Cover the bowl with a sheet of transparent paper and leave to

marinate for 30 minutes.

7. After the marinating time, drain the tofu and place it in a pan brushed with olive oil.

8. Sprinkle the tofu with the filtered marinating liquid and cook in the oven for 10 minutes at 200 ° C.

9. As soon as 10 minutes have passed, take the tofu out of the oven and make it into slices.

10. Put it on serving plates, sprinkle with the cooking juices and serve.

Tofu with peas and tomato

PREPARATION TIME: 20 minutes

COOKING TIME: 15 minutes
CALORIES: 212

INGREDIENTS FOR 4 SERVINGS

- 400 grams of tofu
- 200 grams of peas
- 250 grams of cherry tomatoes
- 1 shallot
- Olive oil to taste
- Salt and pepper to taste

DIRECTIONS

1. Rinse the tofu, pat it dry with absorbent paper and then cut it into cubes.
2. Rinse the peas and let them drain.
3. Wash the cherry tomatoes and then cut them in half.
4. Peel and wash the shallot, then cut it into slices.
5. Put a tablespoon of oil in a pan and when it is hot enough, put the shallot to brown.
6. Cook for a couple of minutes and then add the cherry tomatoes.
7. Stir and cook for 5 minutes.
8. Now add the peas and continue cooking, stirring occasionally, for another 5 minutes.
9. Now add the tofu and half a glass of water and continue to cook

for another 5 minutes.

10. Season with salt and pepper, stir and then turn off.

11. Put the tofu and vegetables on plates, sprinkled with the cooking juices, and serve.

Tofu with tomato and tzatziki sauce

PREPARATION TIME: 20 minutes
COOKING TIME: 15 minutes
CALORIES: 270

INGREDIENTS FOR 4 SERVINGS

- 400 grams of tofu
- 250 grams of cherry tomatoes
- 100 grams of homemade tzatziki sauce (see basic recipe)
- 1 shallot
- Olive oil to taste
- Salt and pepper to taste

DIRECTIONS

1. Rinse the tofu, pat it dry with a paper towel and then cut it into cubes.
2. Wash the cherry tomatoes and then cut them in half.
3. Peel and wash the shallot, then cut it into slices.
4. Put a tablespoon of oil in a pan and when it is hot enough, put the shallot to brown.
5. Cook for a couple of minutes and then add the cherry tomatoes.
6. Stir and cook for 5 minutes.
7. Now add the tofu and half a glass of water and continue to cook for another 5 minutes.
8. Season with salt and pepper, stir and then turn off.

9. Put the tofu and vegetables on plates, sprinkled with the cooking juices, and tzatziki sauce.
10. You can serve.

Quiche with radicchio

PREPARATION TIME: 20 minutes
COOKING TIME: 20 minutes
CALORIES: 513

INGREDIENTS FOR 4 SERVINGS

- 300 grams of plant based puff pastry
- 2 radicchio
- 450 grams of plant based ricotta
- 3 teaspoons of honey
- 10 chopped walnuts
- 1 teaspoon of nutmeg
- Olive oil to taste
- Salt and pepper to taste

DIRECTIONS

1. Wash the radicchio and then cut the leaves into small pieces.
2. Brown the radicchio in a pan with two tablespoons of olive oil.
3. As soon as the radicchio has changed colour, add the honey, salt and pepper.
4. Mix well to flavour everything.
5. As soon as the honey has melted, turn off.
6. In a bowl put the ricotta, salt, pepper and nutmeg. Mix everything well until you get a smooth cream.
7. Now add the walnuts and mix again.
8. Brush a pan with olive oil and then line it with the puff pastry.

9. Put the ricotta mixture inside.

10. Now put the pastry in the oven and cook at 180°C for 20 minutes.

11. As soon as it is cooked, take it out of the oven and decorate it with radicchio.

12. Cut it into slices, put it on plates and serve.

Carrot quiche

PREPARATION TIME: 20 minutes
COOKING TIME: 50 minutes
CALORIES: 333

INGREDIENTS FOR 4 SERVINGS

- 300 grams of plant based puff pastry
- 500 grams of carrots
- 1 clove of garlic
- 1 teaspoon of chopped chives
- 50 ml of soymilk
- Olive oil to taste
- Salt and pepper to taste

DIRECTIONS

1. Peel and wash the carrots. Cook the carrots in abundant salted water for 10 minutes.
2. As soon as they are cooked, drain them and then cut them into slices.
3. Meanwhile, peel the garlic, wash it and chop it.
4. Heat a tablespoon of olive oil in a pan and as soon as it is hot, brown.
5. Now add the carrots and sauté them for 3 minutes.
6. Season with salt and pepper, mix and turn off. Add the milk and chives and mix again.
7. Take a baking tray and brush it with olive oil.

8. Line the pan with the puff pastry.

9. Put the carrots inside and put in the oven.

10. Cook at 180 ° C for 40 minutes.

11. As soon as it is cooked, remove from the oven and let it cool.

12. Cut the quiche into slices, put it on plates and serve.

Quiche with spinach, pumpkin and tofu

PREPARATION TIME: 20 minutes
COOKING TIME: 70 minutes
CALORIES: 368

INGREDIENTS FOR 4 SERVINGS

- 400 grams of pumpkin
- 300 grams of plant based puff pastry
- 200 grams of spinach
- 1 clove of garlic
- 1 shallot
- 100 grams of tofu
- Olive oil to taste
- Salt and pepper to taste

DIRECTIONS

1. Peel and wash the garlic and shallots, then chop them.
2. Peel the pumpkin, remove the seeds, wash it and cut it into cubes.
3. Wash the spinach and then let it drain.
4. Rinse and then blot with absorbent paper.
5. Bring a pot of water and salt to a boil and then boil the spinach for 5 minutes.
6. Put a tablespoon of olive oil in a pan and as soon as it is hot, brown the garlic and shallots.
7. As soon as they are golden, add the pumpkin.

8. Season with salt and pepper, stir and then add half a glass of water.

9. Cook for 10 minutes then turn off.

10. Brush a pan with olive oil and then line it with the puff pastry.

11. Put the pumpkin inside first and then the spinach.

12. Crumble the tofu over the vegetables with your hands.

13. Put in the oven and cook for 40 minutes at 190 ° C.

14. As soon as it is cooked, take it out of the oven, let it rest for 10 minutes and then cut it into slices.

15. Put on serving plates and serve.

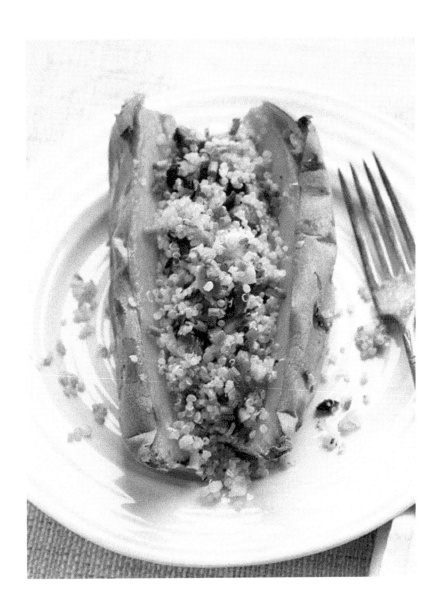

Chickpea and vegetable burgers

PREPARATION TIME: 20 minutes
COOKING TIME: 40 minutes
CALORIES: 351

INGREDIENTS FOR 4 SERVINGS

- 4 wholemeal hamburger buns

- 100 grams of cooked chickpeas

- 1 potato

- 1 carrot

- wholemeal breadcrumbs

- 1 onion

- 16 cherry tomatoes

- 4 lettuce leaves

- 4 teaspoons of vegan mayonnaise

- olive oil to taste

- salt and pepper to taste

DIRECTIONS

1. Wash the potato with all the peel and then boil it in salted boiling water for 20 minutes.

2. When it is ready, drain it, pass it under running water and peel it.

3. Put the chickpeas in the potato scraper and mash them in a bowl.

4. Do the same with the potato.

5. Peel the carrot, wash it and chop it. Put it in the bowl with the vegetables.

6. Mix and then add the breadcrumbs.

7. Season with salt and pepper and mix again.

8. Now form four large meatballs with the mixture and then mash them.

9. Pass them on a plate with breadcrumbs.

10. Brush a baking sheet with olive oil and then lay the burgers inside.

11. Sprinkle them with a little oil and cook them in the oven at 180 ° c for 20 minutes.

12. Take the burgers out of the oven and let them rest.

13. In the meantime, wash the cherry tomatoes and cut them into slices.

14. Wash and dry the lettuce leaves.

15. Cut the burger buns in half and brush the mayonnaise.

16. Put the tomato, the burger and finally the lettuce and close the buns.

17. You can serve.

Mushrooms with tofu and tomatoes

PREPARATION TIME: 25 minutes
CALORIES: 243

INGREDIENTS FOR 4 SERVINGS

- 500 grams of Champignon mushrooms
- 2 tablespoons of lemon juice
- 120 grams of tofu
- 2 tomatoes
- 1 teaspoon of dried oregano
- Salt and pepper to taste
- Olive oil to taste

DIRECTIONS

1. Wash the tomatoes, cut them in half and remove seeds and pulp.
2. Collect the seeds and pulp in a bowl.
3. Cut the tomatoes into thin slices.
4. Remove the earthy part of the mushrooms, wash them, dry them and cut them into slices.
5. Dab the tofu with absorbent paper and then grill it for 3 minutes per side.
6. When it is ready, put it on a slicer and cut it into cubes.
7. Prepare the sauce. In the bowl with the pulp of the tomatoes put oil, salt, pepper and lemon juice. Mix well with a fork.
8. Now put the mushrooms on a serving dish put the tomatoes and grilled tofu on top and sprinkle with the sauce.
9. Sprinkle with oregano and serve.

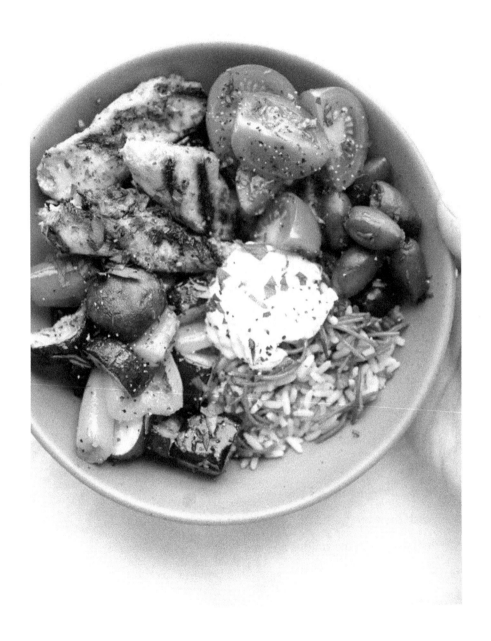

Gratin of seitan and vegetables

PREPARATION TIME: 20 minutes
COOKING TIME: 50 minutes
CALORIES: 212

INGREDIENTS FOR 4 SERVINGS

- 200 grams of seitan

- 2 medium sized potatoes

- 6 tomatoes

- 2 onions

- 200 ml of vegetable broth

- Olive oil to taste

- Salt and pepper to taste

DIRECTIONS

1. Wash the potatoes with all the peel and put them to cook in a pot with boiling water and salt for 25 minutes.

2. Drain the potatoes, pass them under cold water and then peel them.

3. Now cut them into slices.

4. Wash the tomatoes and then cut them into slices.

5. Peel and wash the onions and then cut them into slices.

6. Heat a tablespoon of oil in a pan and brown the onion for 5 minutes. Season with salt and pepper and turn off.

7. Dab the seitan with absorbent paper and then cut it into strips.

8. Now put the seitan in the pan with the onions.

9. Cook for 5 minutes and then turn off.

10. Brush a baking dish with olive oil and put a layer of potatoes at the bottom. Season them with oil, salt and pepper.

11. Put the onions and seitan on top and a layer of tomatoes on top. Also, season the tomatoes with oil, salt and pepper.

12. Continue until you have used up all the ingredients.

13. Pour the vegetable broth over the vegetables and bake for 20 minutes at 180 °.

14. Just cooked, take it out of the oven, let it rest for 5 minutes and then serve directly in the baking dish.

Tempeh stew with oranges and olives

PREPARATION TIME: 10 minutes
COOKING TIME: 20 minutes
CALORIES: 370

INGREDIENTS FOR 4 SERVINGS

- 400 grams of tempeh

- 2 oranges

- 16 black olives

- 1 red onion

- 250 ml of vegetable broth

- a tablespoon of chopped chives

- oat flour to taste

- olive oil to taste

- salt and pepper to taste

DIRECTIONS

1. Wash the oranges, grate the zest of one orange and squeeze the juice of the other two into a bowl.

2. Dab the tempeh with paper towel and then cut it into cubes.

3. Put the oatmeal on a plate and then flour the tempeh.

4. Peel and wash the onion and then chop it.

5. Heat a tablespoon of oil in a saucepan and when hot, sauté the tempeh for a couple of minutes.

6. Add the onion and chives, season with salt, pepper, and sauté for 3 minutes.

7. Now add the broth and orange juice and bring to a boil.

8. At this point, turn off and add the orange zest.

9. Stir, put on plates and serve.

Spicy seitan stew

PREPARATION TIME: 10 minutes
COOKING TIME: 20 minutes
CALORIES: 340

INGREDIENTS FOR 4 SERVINGS

- 400 grams of seitan

- 1 carrot

- 1 stick of celery

- 1 onion

- 300 ml of vegetable broth

- white pepper to taste

- a pinch nutmeg

- a teaspoon of grated ginger

- oat flour to taste

- olive oil to taste

- salt to taste

DIRECTIONS

1. Peel and wash the carrot then chop it.

2. Wash the celery and then chop it.

3. Peel and wash the onion and then chop it.

4. Rinse and pat the seitan with absorbent paper and then cut it into cubes.

5. Put the oatmeal on a plate and then flour the seitan cubes.

6. Put a tablespoon of olive oil in a saucepan and as soon as it is hot, add the carrot, onion and celery to sauté for 2 minutes.

7. Add the seitan cubes and mix well.

8. Now add the salt and all the spices and mix again.

9. Now add the vegetable broth and cook for 10 minutes, stirring occasionally.

10. After the cooking time, turn off, put on plates and serve.

Seitan slices with pistachios and cherry tomatoes

PREPARATION TIME: 10 minutes
COOKING TIME: 10 minutes
CALORIES: 376

INGREDIENTS FOR 4 SERVINGS

- 400 grams of seitan

- 1 shallot

- 100 grams of chopped pistachios

- 12 cherry tomatoes

- Oat flour to taste

- Salt and pepper to taste

- Olive oil to taste

DIRECTIONS

1 Dab the seitan with absorbent paper and then cut it into slices.

2 Put the oatmeal on a plate and flour the seitan slices on both sides.

3 Wash the cherry tomatoes and then cut them in half.

4 Put a tablespoon of olive oil in a pan and as soon as it is hot, put the slices of seitan to cook.

5 Brown them for 3 minutes on each side, then remove, and set aside.

6 Now put the pistachios and cherry tomatoes in the pan.

7 Mix well and cook for 5 minutes.

8 Now put the seitan slices again and season with salt and pepper.

9 Cook for a couple of minutes and then turn off.

10 Put the slices on the plates; surround them with the cherry tomatoes.

11 Sprinkle everything with the cooking sauce and serve.

Tofu and figs salad

PREPARATION TIME: 10 minutes
COOKING TIME: 5 minutes
CALORIES: 180

INGREDIENTS FOR 4 SERVINGS

- 100 grams of tofu

- 4 figs

- 400 grams of mixed green salad

- Olive oil to taste

- Salt and pepper to taste

- Balsamic vinegar to taste

DIRECTIONS

1   Wash and dry the green salad.

2   Wash and dry the figs and then cut them into four wedges.

3   Dab the tofu and then cut it into cubes.

4   Heat a tablespoon of olive oil in a pan and then cook the tofu for 5 minutes.

5   Put the mixed salad on the bottom of a salad bowl.

6   Place the figs and tofu on top.

7   Season with oil, salt, pepper and balsamic vinegar and then serve.

Peas and tofu mousse

PREPARATION TIME: 10 minutes
COOKING TIME: 25 minutes
CALORIES: 210

INGREDIENTS FOR 4 SERVINGS

- 300 grams of shelled peas
- 1shallot
- 100 grams of tofu
- 200 ml of vegetable broth
- A sprigs of thyme
- Olive oil to taste
- Salt and pepper to taste

DIRECTIONS

1. Peel and wash the shallot and then chop it.
2. Wash and dry the thyme sprigs.
3. Rinse the peas and let them drain.
4. Heat a tablespoon of oil in a saucepan and put the shallot to fry for 2 minutes.
5. Add the peas and mix. Season with salt and pepper and then add the vegetable broth.
6. Cook for 20 minutes.
7. Meanwhile, rinse and pat the tofu and then cut it into small pieces.

8. After 20 minutes, put the tofu and the chopped thyme in the pot with the peas.

9. Cook for 5 minutes, and then turn off.

10. Take an immersion blender and blend everything.

11. Put in a bowl and the mousse is ready to be served.

Baked tofu

PREPARATION TIME: 10 minutes
COOKING TIME: 15 minutes
CALORIES: 298

INGREDIENTS FOR 4 SERVINGS

- 200 grams of tofu
- 1 red onion
- 12 cherry tomatoes
- 20 black olives
- A teaspoon of dried oregano
- Olive oil to taste
- Salt and pepper to taste

DIRECTIONS

1   Wash the cherry tomatoes and then cut them into 4 wedges.

2   Peel and wash the onion and then cut it into thin slices.

3   Rinse the tofu and then pat it dry with absorbent paper.

4   Brush a baking sheet with olive oil.

5   Place the tofu in the centre of the baking sheet.

6   Now put the onion, the cherry tomatoes and the olives.

7   Season everything with oil, salt and pepper and then sprinkle with oregano.

8   Bake in the oven at 200 ° C for 15 minutes.

9   As soon as it is ready, take out of the oven, put the tofu and vegetables on a serving dish and serve.

Tofu with balsamic vinegar and pistachios

PREPARATION TIME: 10 minutes
COOKING TIME: 10 minutes
CALORIES: 214

INGREDIENTS FOR 4 SERVINGS

* 200 grams of tofu
*
* 1 tablespoon of soy sauce
* 2 tablespoons of balsamic vinegar
* 1 garlic clove
* 2 tablespoons of chopped pistachios
* Olive oil to taste
* Salt and pepper to taste

DIRECTIONS

1. Put the soy sauce, 2 tablespoons of olive oil and the balsamic vinegar in a bowl. With a fork, mix and emulsify well.
2. Peel and wash the garlic and then chop it.
3. Put the garlic, salt and pepper in the bowl with the emulsion.
4. Rinse the tofu and then pat it dry with paper towel.
5. Brush a pan with olive oil and place the tofu in the centre of the pan.
6. Sprinkle the tofu with the emulsion.
7. Put in the oven and cook at 180º C for 10 minutes.
8. After 10 minutes, take the tofu out of the oven and place it on a serving dish.
9. Sprinkle with the chopped pistachios and put on the table.

Tofu chunks with flax seeds and soy sauce

PREPARATION TIME: 10 minutes
COOKING TIME: 10 minutes
CALORIES: 214

INGREDIENTS FOR 4 SERVINGS

- 400 grams of tofu
- 4 tablespoons of flax seeds
- 80 ml tablespoons of soy sauce
- Olive oil to taste
- pepper to taste

DIRECTIONS

1. Rinse the tofu, pat it dry with absorbent paper and then cut it into cubes.
2. Put the flax seeds on a plate and then pass over the tofu cubes.
3. Heat two tablespoons of oil in a pan and when hot, sauté the tofu.
4. Sauté for a couple of minutes and then add the soy sauce.
5. Cook until the soy sauce has thickened slightly.
6. At this point turn off, season with a little pepper and mix.
7. Put the tofu cubes on the plates, sprinkle them with the cooking juices and serve.

Stracchino baked carrots

PREPARATION TIME: 15 minutes

COOKING TIME: 20/25 minutes
CALORIES: 296

INGREDIENTS FOR 4 SERVINGS

- 800 grams of carrots

- 180 grams of plant-based stracchino (see basic recipe)

- 100 ml of soymilk cream

- 1 shallot

- Olive oil to taste

- Salt and pepper to taste

DIRECTIONS

1. Peel the carrots and then wash them. Cut them into thin slices.

2. Peel and wash the shallot and then chop it.

3. Put two tablespoons of olive oil in a pan and as soon as it is hot, put the shallot to brown.

4. After a couple of minutes, add the carrots.

5. Season with salt and pepper, stir and let them cook for 10 minutes.

6. Meanwhile, put the stracchino and cream in a bowl.

7. Add salt, pepper and mix well.

8. Brush a pan with olive oil and then put the carrots inside.

9. Sprinkle them with the stracchino mixture and put them in the oven.

10. Cook at 220 ° C for 20 minutes.

11. After 20 minutes, check the cooking and if they are not yet golden on the surface, continue cooking for another 5 minutes.
12. As soon as they are cooked, take them out of the oven; let them rest for 2 minutes.
13. Put on serving plates and serve.

I hope this guide will help you and that it can somehow help you to have better health, and to lose weight while staying fit.

Carolyn J. Perez

Lightning Source UK Ltd.
Milton Keynes UK
UKHW050014280521
384471UK00010BA/779